My Journey vs Chronic Fibromyalgia & Treating It

Shannon Donaldson

Legal Disclaimer

The information contained in this eBook is offered for informational purposes solely, and it is geared towards providing exact and reliable information in regards to the topic and issue covered. Also, this eBook provides information only up to the publishing date.

The author and the publisher does not warrant that the information contained in this e-book is fully complete and shall not be responsible for any errors or omissions. The author and publisher shall have neither liability nor responsibility to any person or entity concerning any reparation, damages, or monetary loss caused or alleged to be caused directly or indirectly by this e-book. Therefore, this eBook should be used as a guide - not as the ultimate source.

The publication is sold with the idea that the publisher is not required to render accounting, officially permitted, or otherwise, qualified services. If advice is necessary, legal or professional, a practiced individual in the profession should be ordered.

- From a Declaration of Principles which was accepted and approved equally by a Committee of Publishers and Associations:

Table of Content

Legal Disclaimer

Table of Content

Chapter 1 - An Overview of Fibromyalgia

What is Fibromyalgia? 7

Impact On Daily Life 11

Chapter 2 - Stressors of Fibromyalgia

Symptoms and Health Problems Caused by Stress ..16

Possible Ways To Ease Everyday Stressors...............17

Chapter 3 - Fibrofog

What Are Some of the Causes of Fibrofog? 24

Chapter 4 - After The Doctor's Recommendation

More Information about Fibromyalgia.....................29

Chapter 5 - Fibromyalgia And Pain Hypersensitivity

The 18 Fibromyalgia Tender Points..........................31

Chapter 6 - Treating the Aches

Medical Treatments Vs. Holistic Treatments 36

Going the Holistic Way 38

Acupuncture 40

Using The Marijuana Plant for the Pain Caused by Fibromyalgia 41

Chapter 7 - Deep Relaxation Techniques

Meditation..45

Massage...46

Yoga 47

Chapter 8 - Depression And Anxiety - The Fibromyalgia Connection

How Depression Affects Fibromyalgia......................49

Chapter 9 - Other Diseases Similar to Fibromyalgia

Chronic Fatigue Syndrome and Fibromyalgia...........50

Similarities Between CFS and Fibromyalgia Syndrome51

Differences between CFS and FM 52

Know Your Illness 53

Chapter 10 - Food And Diet

What are the Ideal Solutions? 54

Chapter 11 - Using Herbal & Mental Detox To Treat Fibromyalgia

Detox for Overall Healing 57

The Digestive System..58

Food Sensitivities...59

Conclusion: Living With Fibromyalgia

Chapter 1 - An Overview of Fibromyalgia

As I started writing this book I would simply forget what I was writing. I would forget that I was even writing a book, yet what the book was about. But yet, I have managed to finish writing this book. So what is this book about some may ask. Well this book is about how I deal with my life's journey versus Fibromyalgia. It contains a few tricks and tips that I use to get a better handle on this chronic disease, Fibromyalgia.

What is Fibromyalgia?

I can tell you what Fibromyalgia is not. It is not contagious, thank God. It is not just a mind thing. It is Real. So real that the pain can be debilitating. It can be specific to an area of the body and cause great pain. Excruciating pain or a dull stiff pain. Especially early in the morning. Some days I have to get up early to start my day. So that I may adjust to the stiffness and any other morning aches that will subdue by late afternoon.

Fibromyalgia is a chronic condition, however you cannot die from it. But you will have pain forever, if not routinely taken care of. It can be characterised by a wide range of symptoms. Including stiffness, and tenderness of the muscles, tendons, and joints. The symptoms may be constant or intermittent for years or even an lifetime.

One time I vomited for 6 months, non-stop every day. The doctors ran every test that they could think of. There was no explanation for it. I was constantly vomiting each and every single day for 6 months straight. It was just the weirdest thing. Another time I had chronic hives for another 6 months. I couldn't even touch my own skin without a group of hives popping up. I took all kinds of allergy pills and sensitive fabric detergent. Nothing truly seemed to help soothe my aches. One day it just magically stopped.

Unfortunately the primary symptom of Fibromyalgia is found in other disorders so getting a proper diagnosis is more challenging. It is a widespread and diffused pain, often including needlelike tingling of the skin, the ache in the muscles, weakness in the limb, and pain in the nerves. The tingling is like no other.

A good example that I can think of is when you are sitting at a desk for too long. Your leg may as we say, fall asleep. It feels tingly. If you shake your leg, apply pressure or stand up to help increase circulation it feels better. Well not with Fibromyalgia.

On a good night the tingling may last for 4 hours. Can you imagine you're feeling so numb and tingly for hours? For me it seems to happen more at night then during the day time. I try to help treat the tingling as soon as I feel it. No need to be uncomfortable for hours. I do leg stretches and do basic yoga. I take it back to elementary school days being in the gym with all of your friends. Stretching before a game of dodge ball. Honestly those basic stretches does the job.

For myself, fibromyalgia flare up can be random sometimes. I feel as though my flare ups are based on how my body is feeling. For example, lack of deep sleep, exhausted from physical activity and from being hungry. I have also noticed that some external factors may cause my Fibromyalgia to flare up. A few of these factors are cold weather, including the air conditioner. Yes the a/c. If I am working at hospital where the air conditioner is constantly blowing cold air on the back of my neck. Oh my, you just don't know. The cold air feels as though it is piercing through my clothes, through my skin and down into the middle of my bones. A cold, shivering, piercing sharp pain. When it rains, it pours. Well for me when it rains, I hurt. The pain can be compared to as Arthritis pain of the joints. But yet, my joints are not inflamed. Weird, right.

Chronic sleep disturbances are also characteristic of Fibromyalgia. It is a condition in which deep sleep is frequently interrupted by burst of brain activity similar to wakefulness. Meaning I can't sleep at night. I wake up tired. Throughout the night my dreams are so vivid that when I wake up I am so exhausted. Yes people dream, but not these kind of dreams. It had gotten to the point that I did not know if I was awoke or dreaming. For my dreams were that vivid.

There was a time when I was out of town on an assignment for work. We were working 12 hour shifts. So I had a daily routine. I would wake up at 5am brush my teeth, get dressed, have a cup of coffee then get on the shuttle for work. I would then work at the hospital for 12 hours, get on the shuttle, go back to the hotel, have dinner, get ready for bed and then sleep. Well in my very vivid dream, I was doing the exact same routine. So I didn't know if I was awoke or just dreaming. Did I even go to sleep? How much sleep did I get? Am I still dreaming right now? I felt like I was in the movie Inception. I cried when I first had watched that movie, for I felt that was me trapped in a dream. I somehow got through it after a couple of weeks things finally went back to normal.

If I do not get 8 hours of sleep on a consistent basis I flare up. It is just that simple. I have found that it doesn't matter what symptoms may be showing its ugly face, sleep does the job. Sleep is my best friend, ever since the symptom chronic fatigue took over me. I have grown to love sleep. No on a serious note, when in a flare up sleep helps rejuvenate my body. It calms the flare up down. Chronic fatigue is whole another beast. One time I had chronic fatigue for 2 ½ days. I was so fatigue I slept all day and all night. No food and no bathroom break. I didn't even change positions in the bed. I couldn't hold my head up. Around the 3rd day I had more energy to get up. I wasn't all the way myself until the 4th day.

One more trigger for me is Stress.

Impact On Daily Life

It may be reassuring to know, however, that fibromyalgia isn't life-threatening. Fibromyalgia does not harm your muscles, joints, or organs, plus there are many things you can do to control it. Fibromyalgia is more common in relatives of patients' who suffer from it, suggesting the contribution of both genetic and environmental factors.

Though not fatal, Fibromyalgia can affect every aspect of one's life. It can severely curtail the recreation and social activity. Medical report shows around 30% of the Fibromyalgia are unable to maintain their job. A person with this disease should know as much about the syndromes, symptoms, and treatments as they can. So that they can fully participate in the long course of Fibromyalgia treatment.

Becoming educated about Fibromyalgia gives the person more potential for improvement. Fibromyalgia can be managed, but it needs to be managed differently than a standard disease. Fibromyalgia is a debilitating syndrome that is often associated with impaired cellular energy metabolism.

Chapter 2 - Stressors of Fibromyalgia

I believe that I did not learn how to properly express my emotions and how to deal with stress. I tend to out of sight, out mind it. I didn't deal with a problem that was causing the stress head on. I kept it inside and to myself. I didn't properly digest it. So in return for me my emotions wore my body as Fibromyalgia. My stress manifests itself as Fibromyalgia. For it is a reflection of emotional and physical stress which in turn increases pain and fatigue, thus creating more stress.

If I get upset, I flare up. If I am sad, I flare up. If someone pokes me, pinch me, hit me or squeeze me. Then I flare up. If I get too excited, overly happy with excitement. I flare up. Bad news put me down for a week or more. And when I say I flare up, I mean my trigger points are lightening up. I am having muscle spasms in my neck muscles, shoulders, upper right back, lower back, shooting pain down my legs. Down to my toes and the arch of my foot will start spazzing. My whole arm hurts, the muscles around my elbow is hurting differently from the pain in my forearm. Which is a different pain from my wrist. Then each and every single finger hurt at each and every joint with the surrounding connective tissue. And when that happens, I cannot use my arms. I prop myself up on my full length body pillow with the heating pad. I have the heating pad positioned to my neck, shoulders and upper back. For that hurts the most and the heat helps soothe the aches. I at times may rotate with an ice pack. I know cold makes me hurt. But depending on where the pain is, that icepack does the job. Such as isolated pain at the back of my head, the occipital. The icepack is very ideal for that kind of pain. It's not a headache, it is a pain in the head.

Stress affects your body as much as food and exercise. Some stress is good stress. It can cause a boost in energy. It can push you to do your best. Then there is the bad stress. Any prolonged stress weakens a person over time leaving them wide open and susceptible to even more stress both physically and emotionally.

The Oxford Dictionary defines the word "stress" as "a state of an affair involving demand on physical or mental energy".

This demand on the mind-body occurs when it tries to cope with continual changes in life. In moderation, stress is a normal part of life and in many cases, proves useful, but extreme stress is detrimental to human health and creates an excellent breeding ground for illness. Stress is also a common precursor of psychological difficulties such as anxiety and depression.

Too much stress for too long becomes distressed and this is where the problems lie. Distress results when our bodies overreact to events. Each person has their degree of tolerance in how they react or handle stress or stressful events. Some people handle stress well, and it has little impact on their physical or emotional health while others are very negatively influenced by it. Lifestyle factors very much influence our ability to cope or deal with stress. Lack of sleep, inadequate or improper nutrition and diet, and excessive alcohol consumption and smoking can all put more stress on the body while at the same time they lower our tolerance or ability to handle stress.

Other sources of stress include personal relationships, family, traffic, workplace, noise, meeting deadlines, cold temperature, pain, or accidents. Even life changing events suchs as jobs, the birth of a new baby and moving are all forms of stress. A lot of people tend to worry a lot. They worry over everything. I had to learn patience, when dealing with Fibromylgia. And to not worry. God will handle it.

Symptoms and Health Problems Caused by Stress

Stress can cause the following symptoms and health problems:

— Fatigue
— Headaches
— Insomnia or other changes in sleep patterns
— Memory loss
— Nightmares
— Mood changes or swings
— Accident Prone
— Loss of enthusiasm or no motivation to do anything
— Crying spells
— Lack of focus, can't concentrate
— Gastrointestinal disorders
— Allergies
— Skin rashes, or irritations
— Asthma
— Diarrhea or constipation

— Changes in appetite
— Teeth-grinding
— Cold hands
— Sweaty palms
— Shallow breathing
— Nervous twitches
— High blood pressure
— Lowered sexual drive
— Low self-esteem
— Depression

Although Fibromyalgia has been linked to several stressful or traumatic events, other possible causes include physical or emotional trauma, infection/virus, co-morbid conditions that eventually trigger fibromyalgia, cervical stenosis, abnormal pain response, genetic predisposition, etc.

Possible Ways To Ease Everyday Stressors

Theses are a few tips that I use to avoid stress.

1. **Get a good understanding of the illness.** This will go a long way toward accepting it and creating a positive mental outlook and a plan to conquer Fibromyalgia.

2. **Learn to read your body**. Many people living with chronic pain learn to ignore what their body is saying as a means of coping. It is preferable to learn to recognize signs of stress and tension such as a headache, shoulder tension, clenching jaw and heartburn. Recognize what contributes to the flare up.

3. **Change the way you react to situations**. Patience, patience, patience will help me in the long term. This involves me looking at a situation from all angles. From various points of views. Many situations are outside of my control, so taking it upon myself and allowing it to affect me is pointless. When it is all said and done I will be the one suffering from pain. So why hold onto things that are unhealthy for me.

4. **Good Self-care is essential to overall well being and reducing stress.** This involves a good, healthy

diet, the proper exercise, giving yourself permission to rest when needed, and developing good sleep habits are all important aspects of a healthy lifestyle.

5. **Learn to say NO**. Often people with Fibromyalgia have a difficult time learning the balance between wanting to be able to do things and actually being able to do those things. At times taking one for the team is not ideal. For you will be the one to suffer alone later. There are moments when I had felt guilty because I feel that I should be more active. It seems as though I always have an excuse on why I can not make it to a function. Then on other days I am out and about alone. On my own terms.

There are several other methods you can use to combat stress, including physiotherapy and massage therapy, meditation, deep breathing exercises, progressive muscle relaxation, mental imagery relaxation, relaxation to music, biofeedback, counseling - to help you recognize and release stress. Also, you can learn stress management techniques and if necessary, talk to a counselor who specialized in stress and pain management.

Chapter 3 - Fibrofog

I started this book by saying that I had forgotten that I was writing a book. So how did I write this book if I had forgotten. Well I would remember the idea of writing a book to help others understand that they are not alone and it can be dealt with and have an almost normal life. But, I would remember over time and through each flare up.

Fibrofog would make me cry. For I don't know which is worst. To be in pain or to not remember. What a lot of people don't know is that for me, that memory never comes back. I have sat and tried over and over to try to remember. I would attempt to retrace my steps, but that would mean that I would have to actually remember my steps. I would then ask a close friend or family member. But then I would just be confused. Or I may not even ask anyone out of embarrassment. For when I ask them, I still do not know what they are talking about. Also I question myself and my actions. I could see me doing something and not remember. To simply do it all over again. Repetitively. It sounds good. But not with me. The next day if you tell my what I did, I may not believe you because I feel as though I wouldn't have done it like that. But yet I did. It's as if I blacked out and became a complete different person. Doing things that I wouldn't normally do while I can remember things. Mind you I am sober and not on any medications. SO why wouldn't I do it the same way twice. Weird, right.

I can remember long term and people. Not so good with names, but who is who. Last night after 8pm may be a blurr to me. Some phone conversations I can not remember. In return I try not to get on the phone with people. With a text message I can replay the conversation and back track so that I know what is going on.

I was taking a herbal supplement, St.John's Wart weekly. There was a point when I didn't know why I was taking these herbal supplements. I knew that it was good for me, but I couldn't remember why I was to take them. One day while reading up on the latest information on Fibromyalgia. I came across the same herbal supplement that I was taking. Apparently it is to help with my memory. Go figure.

One morning I woke up and didn't know who my daughter was. She wasn't even two years old around that time. I had awoken around 9am. I looked over and saw a beautiful little girl. I didn't know who she was. I knew who I was, but not her. I sat there for a few minutes trying to think who's little girl am I watching. Why am I watching this little girl? Is she hungry? Should I change her or let her sleep? HHmm she's really beautiful. Ok no seriously who's little girl is this? Why do I have her? What's going on? Ok calm down, no wait, no calm down I kept telling myself. Don't panic.

I laid back down and started to slowly cry. A little sobbing. Then it hits me that I have no idea what is going on. I just balled my eyes out. I cried myself to sleep. When I woke back up two hours later I could remember everything. Everything including the fact that I couldn't remember and didn't know who my only sweet beautiful child was. I went to the doctor.

Fibrofog is one of the most common symptoms of Fibromyalgia. It is important to be aware of fibrofog so that you can seek appropriate treatment and manage your illness more effectively. It can be very scary and dangerous. Especially if you are consuming an alcoholic beverage while having a a fibrofog flare up.

A few fibrofog symptoms that I have experienced are:
— short-term memory loss
— difficulty remembering where I put things
— difficulty remembering plans
— difficulty holding conversations
— difficulty following conversations
— short attention span during flare ups

— difficulty finding the right word to use in conversation
— slurred words
— trouble with concentrating and focusing

What Are Some of the Causes of Fibrofog?

One symptom my be Sleep deprivation. I'm just not getting enough sleep. I am in pain in my sleep.

If you do not get adequate or quality sleep, it can affect the brain's ability to produce enough of the neurochemical serotonin which aids in laying down memory.

Chronic pain would distract anyone. Imagine your whole body hurting you from each and every single hair root down to your pinky toe. And keep in mind each body hurts differently. All at the same time. I have gotten up from the couch to go use the bathroom. On my way there the arch in my left foot hurts, my right leg is tingling, the muscles between my ribs hurt, my fingers hurt, I can't turn my head to the right completely, my trigger point on mu upper left back is triggering, my lower back hurts, and then there is pain running down my right leg. By the time I got to the bathroom I had forgotten why I was even in there. Now I have to go back to the couch and attempt to try again. Or just let it go.

Chronic pain has been shown to inhibit the brain's ability to create memories. Processing pain signals take up a lot of the brain's time and energy, especially in someone with fibromyalgia. Pain also produces large amounts of stress which can be one of the causes of short-term memory loss.

They say a lot of us who has Fibromyalgia are depressed. I could see how they could think that. For with Fibromyalgia you never know when you may flare up. Which could then result in people becoming anti-social. Withdrawn from others. Limit their activities for out of fear of flaring up. With depression it lowers the levels of serotonin in the brain. With low levels it prevents new memories from being remembered.

Chapter 4 - After The Doctor's Recommendation

After not many years of research, some doctors still have the opinion that this is all in the patient's head, a real disease not being at all present. Genetical en heritage has also been proven to be an important factor in the patient's development of this. So they say

Doctors have decided to take serious action and determine once and for all what makes this illness appear in some people, thus treating patients as normal sick people. They have embarked on a quest to find and learn more about the factors that cause this and this way, if possible, find the best treatments available with modern medicine.

An astonishing number of some 10 million people have been found out to be suffering from this particular and strange Fbromyalgia.

Some doctor's say it's all in your head and ridicule you. There has been several Emergency Room visits where the doctors who didn't specialize in the disease treat me as if I was a drug addict. I must say this, for the record a lot of theses "prescribed" medications DO NOT work. It does not even touch the pain. Time, relaxation and rest helps. I am not going into the ER seeking drugs. I am in need of help and need some relief, for the pain is kicking my ass. That is honesty.

Other Physicians believe that is a neurological disorder, central nervous system disorder. Fight or flight. Well I flare up whether I am overly happy or scared. Then others believe that it is an abnormality of the brain. But is it?

It is the disease that they can not figure out. Doctors have test me during a flare up. The did lab test, endoscopy, bone marrow, research, you name it they did it. Thank God for good health insurance. Not only did they test me for everything, we did a process of elimination on what diseases that it could be.

Then doctors thought that I had lupus. I had tested border line for it. I used to get the butterfly mask across my face when I would go outside in the sun. But my test never went over. It be on a range from 30-100, I would have 29. So therefor, I don't have it. They then thought I had Non-Hodgkin's lymphoma. But my lymphoma nodes weren't swollen. Even through I constantly had chronic laryngitis. Not that it matters just another symptom.

A Physician then sent me to the Infectious Control Disease doctor. I was surrounded by people with HIV and my only test result showed elevated IgE level for allergens. Side note I am allergic to fruits, vegetables and nuts. Other than that my blood work looks like and average healthy person.

I have seen all kinds of doctors and been on all kinds of prescribed medications. I was apart of two research studies on Fibromyalgia. I currently do not take any prescribed medications. I am on a holistic approach. The most I will do is Tramadol, Tylenol, Motrin and Robaxin (muscle relaxer). I go to the sauna on a regular basis, use a heating pad/ice pack, sleep well, Epsom salt, yoga/stretch, massages and use the CBD ointment. One of my doctors had written me a prescription for a medical massage. That way my health insurance would cover the cost. For it can be very costly to go per week or every other week.

Symptoms have been shown to vary a lot in patients: from mild or severe chronic pain throughout the body of the person, to headaches and fatigue and most strangely memory problems and difficulty in concentration.

More Information about Fibromyalgia

Usually, the symptoms of FMS don't come up until a person is an adult. Experts believe that injuries cause the severity of the problem. A stressful stimulus which is administered to the spinal cord can cause this certain problem. Some of the examples of these stressful stimuli are an extended dental work or doing a work which suggests the backbone to be narrowed.

Another interesting finding was revealed. It was found out that women who have undergone breast implant operations have a higher tendency of developing such a condition. This was believed that FMS occurred due to some infections which resulted in the surgery however the research concluded that it was due to the hyperextension of the neck while the patient is under anesthetic.

Usually, people who experience injuries develop FMS. There are a lot of studies which can prove this. It was indicated that 65% of FMS patients developed this condition after an injury. It was then found out that a neck injury is more prone to resulting in FMS than with those who are experienced in the different parts of the body.

Conclusively, further studies are still conducted to find the right answers to a lot of questions that humankind has been asking. With all this being done effective treatments have yet to be found. Still understanding the disease has come a long way from saying it's all in the patient's mind making us believe that the finding of a reliable treatment is just around the corner.

Chapter 5 - Fibromyalgia And Pain Hypersensitivity

The 18 Fibromyalgia Tender Points

Fibromyalgia tender points could be the first warning sign that you have Fibromyalgia (aka, Fibromyalgia Chronic Fatigue Syndrome). Be aware that this sign or symptom is just one of many that you may experience if you have Fibromyalgia. You may have only a few symptoms or a lot of them. Most of the time, the symptoms will overlap, and you will experience several at the same time.

Checking 18 fibromyalgia tender points is the first accepted test that a doctor will perform. Other symptoms you may have will be assessed as well. Because the symptoms vary with each person, your doctor will look at a combination of your symptoms before he will make a concrete diagnosis.

Fibromyalgia Tender points are distributed in four quadrants of the body. You must have experienced pain in 11 of these tender areas for at least three months to be diagnosed with Fibromyalgia Chronic Fatigue Syndrome. Typically, the pain of is spread to six areas:
— Neck
— Shoulders
— Chest
— Hips

— Knees
— Elbows

Although the 18 points are the standard for diagnosis, fibromyalgia research has identified as many as 75 possible tender areas, and they all vary with the individual.

The intensity of the pain in the fibromyalgia tender points may not be as sensitive one day as they are another. Sometimes the tender areas can be so sensitive, that even the slightest touch can cause tremendous pain. You may also experience an all over pain or discomfort called allodynia, along with the fibromyalgia tender points. The four body different sensations you may experience are:

— Tingling
— Achiness
— Muscle spasms
— Limb weakness

Being diagnosed with Fibromyalgia can often have a domino effect, increasing the stress felt on every level, and unless this illness is managed effectively, the stressors multiply over time.

Chapter 6 - Treating the Aches

I believe in order to treat the symptoms you have to have a basic understanding of the signs and symptoms. There are 2 distinct symptoms that a doctor will look for a diagnosis. One of them is chronic pain that is present in all four quadrants of the body and last for several months. Yup, that's me.

The second top symptom is the 18 tender points. A patient must feel pain in 11 or more of the trigger points. These 18 points are the: back of the neck where the base of the skull and neck meets. I wish I could just reach in my skull and apply pressure to ease the pain.

The pain at the front of the neck goes hand in hand with the pain at the back of the neck. The pair is a terrible point. It causes me many missed nights of sleep.

 Recently my muscles around my elbows have been so sore. Feels as if I have been carrying tons of grocery bags at the elbows. I try not to bend at the elbow. My forearms near the crease of my elbow would feel strained.

At first I hadn't realized how much the point in my hips affects me. That pain can just sit on the hips. Or it can radiate and influence other points to trigger. Once loosened up you can real feel the difference. I don't feel so tight up in that area, where the buttocks muscle curves down to the thighs once released.

My lower back does not bother me as other people with Fibromyalgia does. Proper body alignment and stretching can help reduce this tender point. When I do have pain, it is at the top of the buttocks, right at the bottom of the lower back.

 My knees will go out upon ambulating. Sometimes it feels as though it just locks up on me. Behind my knee will get real stiff at times. It mainly goes with the overall morning stiffness. Or even my knee feels wet. Another weird one.

My upper back tender/trigger point goes hand in hand with my neck and shoulders. When one point hurts, normally for me all 3 will hurt. It is the whole back muscles, shoulder blades and neck muscles.

Then there is the chest. My chest may be tender under my collarbone near my ribs. The muscles between my ribs hurt. My sternum/breast bone and the muscles on my sides would feel inflamed. Feels swollen. Feel as though I was hit directly with a baseball bat. Right across my right shoulder blade/neck and beat on my side under my arm. My whole right side of my body is so tense but feels so swollen.

Some areas may hurt more than others.

The Fibromyalgia therapy that I use is more holistic and less invasive. I have tried the different prescribed medications, but honestly it wasn't for me. I felt more sick in other ways due to the side effects. The side effects on top of a flare up did not make me a very happy person. Alternative medicine and holistic techniques have me living a much more painless life.

I use the CBD ointment, heating pad/ice, stretches/basic yoga, massages and the sauna. With the occasional Tramadol, Tylenol, Motrin and Robaxin for the extreme excruciating flare ups.

Medical Treatments Vs. Holistic Treatments

There is no cure for Fibromyalgia. Period
It's symptoms can be managed. Fibromyalgia is in the mind and the body. The brain is connected to the body via the spinal cord. The spinal cord is responsible for a variety

of functions for the body. The spinal cord and the brain are connected through the autonomic nervous system. Neuro messages are transmitted back and forth through the brain and the body. There is a direct relationship between stress and the symptoms. But also with factors such as our environment. I look at Fibromyalgia as a mind and body, dual that needs to be healed.

Think of it as cause and effect. If you hurt me by yelling at me and hurting my feelings. Or by pinching me and causing me physical harm I will cry. I will have a Fibromyalgia flare up within a few minutes my body will take in the cause and process it as some sort of pain. It is truly amazing but, still weird disease.

A women to women example. Every month I have my menstrual cycle. My hormones will go up and down naturally to accommodate for this monthly process. So therefore, I know that I will have two mild flare ups for the month. One right before my monthly cycle. Which may be a little more painful then the flare up after my period. That one is more on the milder side as my hormones shift back around. These two flare ups are a given.

Let's say I have caught a cold. Lord be with me. For I don't just have a regular common cold. My colds tend to mimic the flu once I flare up behind it. I try to take my vitamins weekly. Just to get that extra boost in my immune system. Plus with me being allergic to fresh fruits, vegetables and nuts. I try to get my supplements in for any nutrients that I may be lacking. So far so good. I am not and have not been deficient in any of my nutrients.

Going the Holistic Way

There are some effective therapies that can help you get your life back. There is no remission. Different people respond differently because they have different symptoms and immune systems. My suggestion is to try the least invasive therapy first before going evasive.

I have tried a variety of herbs, essential oils, food and dietary programs, exercises, etc. There are several herbs that you can research. To each it's own. I would recommend consulting with your doctor first before trying anything. I have weird allergies so therefore, I do not try everything. I try to stick with what works. I am also very open to trying new things. As for the herbs, I found that not all of them have worked for me. I do take the

St.John's Wort to help improve my memory. I take a probiotic for my gut. It helps regulate, boost energy, I don't feel so sluggish after taking. And then I take vitamin B complex to help with the fatigue.

My favorite thing that I love to do to help prevent and treat my flare ups is go to the Korean Bathouse. Not just any sauna but Jeju Sauna. It is heaven there. I can address all my needs. I first start off soaking in the mineral hot tub for a good 20 minutes. It helps relax my muscles from head to toe. I then lay under the Red Infrared Light. The energy from the lights penetrates deep beneath the skin and is absorbed by the deep tissues. Which help increases blood flow. Next I get a body shampoo. That is when you are scrubbed from head to toe thoroughly front, back and sides. Then you are rinsed off and a deep tissue or swiss massage is given. You will then receive your choice of facial. Your hair is washed, then one more massage.

After that I do the dry and steam sauna. From there, I go to the other 9 saunas. One is the charcoal sauna for detox, the gold and silver sauna, jade sauna and so forth. Each sauna providing your body with benefits such as flush out impurities, improve circulation, aide in pain and nerve stability. I spend roughly 30 minutes in each of the 8 saunas, because the 9th is the cold room. I go to the cold room last to lock everything in. I spend a maximum of 5 minutes in the cold room. After that I am on cloud 9 for the next 2 weeks. A routine well worth it. I am at ease and at peace while and after visiting this particular sauna.

Acupuncture

Acupuncture and acupressure are also great ways to ease up the pain and the stiffness of your body. This traditional Chinese practice involves inserting thin needles at key points on the body. Acupressure helps in promoting blood circulation, relax your muscles, and stimulate the same pressure points and it may be a good alternative for people who want to avoid needles. It is a great way to overcome the pain of fibromyalgia.

Using The Marijuana Plant for the Pain Caused by Fibromyalgia

Fibromyalgia patients have a lot symptoms, they are required to take just as many drugs, as each drug is designed only to treat one particular symptom. While causing other issues referred to as side effects. Prescribed medications are toxic and can have negative side effects which often add to the pain and frustration.

Medicinal marijuana, on the other hand, can relieve multiple symptoms with one dosage, and with fewer side effects. There are still chemicals that are inhaled when smoking the herb, but some patients find that it does not cause fatigue, and is more effective than other prescribed medications. They claim that it helps to numb the pain and the burning sensations of fibromyalgia. A lot of massage spas are incorporating CBD products into their massage therapy.

The active ingredient in marijuana that helps to relieve the pain and other symptoms is known as delta-9 tetrahydrocannabinol (THC). This compound is put into a drug which helps with sleeping, numbs pain and eases depression. The CBD does not give an euphoric feeling. It alleviates the muscle pain.

Chapter 7 - Deep Relaxation Techniques

Many people with fibromyalgia have sleep problems, including trouble falling asleep or frequent awakenings during the night. I can toss and turn all night for some nights. Once I get a good sleep pattern going I try to maintain it. Sleep disturbance can disturb my whole body.

Some nights my legs are restless. Tingly and painful. That combination is like no other. I try to shake it off but, it just won't shake away. I found that taking Motrin PM at night before bed has been effective with a cup of warm tea and a hot bath. I don't toss as much with this sleep routine. The goal is to achieve deep realm sleep.

Some studies suggest some people with Fibromyalgia will remain in a shallow state of sleep and never experience restful, deep sleep. This will hurt the body. It will slow down the process to repair and replenish itself, rejuvenates itself. Also, poor sleep may make the pain seem worse, and pain can lead to poor sleep. Which will continue the viscous cycle.

Sleep makes me feel better. I feel as though my body rejuvenates itself after a good 8 hours of sleep. I use a full size body pillow. And I have a plush pillow top mattress. I also have a separate memory foam mattress. At times I rotate between mattresses. But, I honestly sleep better on the pillow top mattress. I would suggest that you find you a good mattress that you will feel comfortable and well rested on.

Fatigue and insomnia goes hand and hand.
I personally am not a big fan of sleep aides, well I wasn't. I am now. I use the Motrin PM. A low dose. It helps tame the pain and allows me to not toss and turn as much as night. I do not take it on a regular basis. I only take it during those excruciating flare ups. My daily night routine consist of calming lavender or eucalyptus or spearmint oils, candles or air fresheners. For my night shower or soak I use the same as a body scrub or bath ball. Along with lavender Epsom salt.

Finding a way to get a good night's sleep is a major a key in providing long-term healing and lessening of day to day pain. Sleep truly helps my mind and body.
Getting sufficient sleep around a solid 8 hours, allows the body to heal, reduces muscular stress and provides mental relief from constant pain that occurs continually.

A few other ways that I have tried to induce sleep is with a nice cup of peppermint or chamomile tea. I tend to stay away from the green tea due to it's diuretic properties. The peppermint and chamomile gives a calming and soothing effect. Relaxes the body and warms the mind.

A natural supplement such as melatonin can help one achieve a peaceful sleep. Melatonin is also a natural occurring hormone within in the body that lets it know when it is time to go to sleep. Once you can manage a good night's sleep you can achieve a better manage on the body. It can help combat fatigue which can in return cause more muscle pain and aches.

I also set the tone for bedtime. I turn off laptops/computers and televisions. I play soft classical or gospel music. A warm environment. Then I take a nice hot bath with lavender Epsom salt. The hot steam relaxes me and opens up my pores. Allowing the smell of the eucalypsis and/or spearmint bath bomb to consume me as I relax. This combination will relax the mind and body. Sweat away harmful toxins and promote circulation.

Meditation

Mediatation
A mind/body relaxation technique called biofeedback is designed to do just that. By learning about how their bodies work and learning to control these factors, biofeedback helps individuals learn how to reduce stress.

Deep breathing techniques can help you relax your body and ease your mind.

I use the third eye meditation. It helps relaxes me. It allows me to relax my mind. It can help with stress and anxiety. It allows me to be at peace within myself. I can easily fall asleep while meditating. That's how completely relaxed that I can get.

Massage

I once had a Physician write me a prescription for medical massages. He wanted me to go every week. Which can be quite costly per session. I would need a hour and a half of massage therapy. I found the steam massages were quite effective.

Massage eases stiffness, improves range of motion, reduces pain and helps with stress management.

Fibromyalgia patients commonly suffer from the tightening of the fascia that contributes to pain and muscle fatigue. Myofascial release is a gentle technique that relaxes the fascia and reduces associated pain.

Rubbing, kneading, or stroking all seem to help too. I have brought a hand held massage tool to rub out knots that I can reach. Of course it helps to have someone else rub it out for you. But if you are alone I would truly invest in a hand held massage tool. It will provide some relief.

Yoga

It is easy for people to tell someone with Fibromyalgia to get up and exercise. It is not that simple. I personally do basic yoga such as: cat/cow, mountain pose, downward facing dog, Viparita Karani is my favorite. It help relieves neck and back tension.

When dealing with fibromyalgia, you want to be very careful that you do not over exercise your muscles, as that will only aggravate them even more. There are yoga exercises that are designed for fibromyalgia patients can help to stretch your muscles without aggravating them. These exercises are also very relaxing, and can even help you to fall into a deep sleep at night.

Chapter 8 - Depression And Anxiety - The Fibromyalgia Connection

Nearly a third of people with fibromyalgia also have major depression when they are diagnosed. Many FM sufferers are often made to feel like their pain is "all in their head," but research has consistently proven that Fibromyalgia is not a form of depression or hypochondria. IT IS REAL!

However, there is a connection between FM and other chronic pain conditions for depression and anxiety. Some researchers believe depression may be a result of the chronic pain and fatigue. Others suggest that abnormalities in brain chemistry may lead to both depression and unusual sensitivity to pain. Symptoms of depression may include difficulty concentrating, hopelessness, and loss of interest in favorite activities. Treatment is important because both can make FM worse and interfere with symptom management.

How Depression Affects Fibromyalgia

Depression is a mental illness where you constantly feel sad and have no interest in socializing. It is a constant low mood that interferes with the ability to function and appreciate things in life. It can last for weeks, months, or years.

A few doctors believe that Fibromyalgia is linked to depression. I could see how they may link the two. With constantly being in pain with no relief. No desire to socialize because of embarrassment or fear of a bad flare up out in public. It is a risk that I take going outside each day. I can have a bad flare up at any given time. Any type of flare up whether I am in pain or I am forgetful.

I however, try my hardest each day to not let it get the best of me. I have to be able function each day. Each day is a new challenge that starts over again each day.

Chapter 9 - Other Diseases Similar to Fibromyalgia

Chronic Fatigue Syndrome and Fibromyalgia

Many find it difficult to make a distinction between fibromyalgia, also known as FM, and chronic fatigue syndrome, particularly because the symptoms of both illnesses are very similar. Even doctors and experts, up until now, cannot definitely say if CFS, short for chronic fatigue syndrome, and FM are two different diseases with like symptoms, separate aspects of one disorder, or two completely distinct illnesses.

Chronic fatigue syndrome, on the other hand, is characterized by severe fatigue, experienced during not less than six months. Sufferers of CFS also experience muscle and joint pains, sore throat, non-restive sleep, and general malaise after performing physical activities. Sometimes, especially after a strenuous activity, CFS patients display temporary concentration, cognitive and memory lapses.

Similarities Between CFS and Fibromyalgia Syndrome

As mentioned earlier, the two conditions share quite a number of similar symptoms. If you think you are suffering from one of such illnesses, you need to consult several doctors. A physician whose expertise is in infectious disease might see your symptoms as chronic fatigue syndrome, while a pain and rehabilitation doctor could look at your symptoms as FM.

Most common indications or symptoms of both FM and CFS sufferers are joint and muscular pain, severe fatigue, inability to concentrate, memory lapses, numbness, malaise, and weakness. Meanwhile, clinical likeness of the two includes non-restive sleep or insomnia, lowering of growth hormone and serotonin levels, and diminished blood flow in certain parts of the brain.

Aside from having similar symptoms, both diseases are also more common in women than men. In FMS, women are about eight times more susceptible than men. Both diseases also occur more often in adults than in children.

Differences between CFS and FM

Although patients of both illnesses suffer muscle pain and fatigue, the degree or severity of the two symptoms will help distinguish chronic fatigue syndrome sufferers from fibromyalgia patients. People who experience predominantly debilitating fatigue suffer from CFS, while those whose main symptom is chronic pain in joints and muscles have FM. Another stark difference is that CFS is prompted or initiated by an infectious illness, such as influenza. On the hand, FM is usually triggered by injury, surgery, accident, or a type of physical trauma.

Know Your Illness

The first thing you should do, when diagnosed with either of the two conditions, is to research and learn as much as you can about your condition. It would be easier for you and your doctor to communicate and discuss the disease and possible treatment plans or options, if you have a certain degree of knowledge about the disease. The Internet, local libraries and journals and magazines can help you with learning more about FM and CFS.

Chapter 10 - Food And Diet

Some suggest that people with Fibromyalgia should follow a certain diet. I know that in my case caffeine may cause me to flare up. It is suggested that Fibromyalgia patients should maintain a healthy diet low in fat and high in fiber, with plenty of whole grains, fresh fruits, and vegetables.

If you have looked for a natural cure for fibromyalgia, great results have been had by using the simple approach of changing dietary habits.

If you are on Medication, there is no reason to stop until symptoms have gone. Protein is known as the main issue with fibromyalgia, so as a good start, the recommendation would be to cut back on it significantly.

What are the Ideal Solutions?

1. Ideally, it would be to go vegan, or as close to a plant-based diet as possible. Me personally, I am not built that way. I add more cooked colorful vegetables to my meals.

2. Cut back on gluten and dairy.

3. Cut out, or at least reduce the consumption of all refined sugars, oils, and caffeine, to aid with a natural cure for fibromyalgia.

4. If you are a smoker, stop.

5. Cut back on alcoholic beverages. For me it messes with my memory. Severely.

6. If you eat meat or fish a couple of times a week, eat so in small portions. Eat a variety of meat and not just red meat.

These tips have worked well for many people, with no need for extra medication and with no real extra outlay, except a change of life style. These tips are introduced without much effort. A few simple changes within dietary.

Chapter 11 - Using Herbal & Mental Detox To Treat Fibromyalgia

As the body starts to fill up on healing nutrients the constant inflammation and pain associated with fibromyalgia will decrease. Unsalted beans should also be consumed daily along with a few tablespoons of raw healthy seeds such as sesame, flax, and pumpkin. So suggested. My family is Jamaican. I eat my beans with my rice.

Detox for Overall Healing

Detox includes various fasting techniques, colonics, enemas, ingesting different herbal compounds or supplements to "cleanse" the body and rid it of all toxins. I however use the sauna for detoxing.

I suggest to have a clean out all of the toxins (heavy metals, xenoestrogens, chemical residues, etc.) that are poisoning your body. Especially with women and the hormonal changes.

It is a must to provide all of the systems and cells in your body with the nutrients they require (vitamins, minerals, trace minerals, antioxidants, phytochemicals, etc.) for optimum vitality and regeneration.

The idea behind detox for Fibromyalgia is relatively simple – Be aware of what to put into your body and be aware of what to avoid. The most important thing to encourage a Fibromyalgia detox begins with a combination of herbs brewed into a tea to remove toxins from your body.

These herbs include Echinacea, fenugreek, and ginger. Brewed together into a tea, these herbs with honey as a sweetener will begin a natural detox when consumed daily. I personally take the Echinacea supplements.

The Digestive System

Fibromyalgia is said to be an autoimmune disorder. It is important to have a healthy body. It is a must to protect the body from bad bacteria that could cause a flare up.
The reason the digestive system (referred to as the gut) is so important is because 70% of your immune system lives just under the surface of your intestinal lining, and any disruption in the beneficial bacteria (lactobacilli, bifidobacteria, those good bugs in yogurt, or the intestinal lining), will cause immune reactions that release inflammatory molecules that travel throughout the body causing inflammation at distant sites. I take a probiotic on a regular basis. Now a days you can find probiotics as a supplement pill, powder, energy bar or as a drink.

Fixing the gut can sometimes completely relieve pain and inflammation in the muscles and joints. A leaky gut could make anyone sick. For myself I have had issues with improperly digesting food. I can only eat small meals at a time. My stomach takes longer to digest food than others.

I would suggest to look for signs of a dysbiosis, an overgrowth of "bad" bacteria, yeast, and/or parasites, signs of leaky gut syndrome, a condition where there is increased permeability in the intestinal lining. These conditions can cause distant inflammation and have been implicated in fibromyalgia, arthritis, and autoimmune disease. Once suspected it can be treated with herbs and supplements that restore health of the digestive tract. Again consult with your physician.

Food Sensitivities

Fibromyalgia has been linked to the "leaky gut" syndrome.

I have personally had my share of gut issues. I take a probiotic on a regular basis. It helps rid of the bad bacteria and promotes the healthy bacteria that is supposed to be there. What exactly is a "leaky gut" you may ask. Well without a good intestinal barrier, a "leaky gut" allows partially digested food to get into the bloodstream. Once that happens then a systemic inflammatory reaction results in painful muscles, joints, or tendons, and also fatigue and "brain fog." To treat this form fibromyalgia, most people will need to eliminate certain foods from their diet while the leaky gut is being treated.

Over the years my list foods that I am allergic to grew. At first it was just a banana that I couldn't eat. Then it was a banana and an apple. Then all of a sudden I couldn't have a salad. And I used to love salads. I would make a fruit salad with apples, bananas, pears, walnuts and whip cream. Now I can only look at it and not touch. However, if the vegetables are cooked and the fruits are baked. Interesting fact, when I was pregnant with my daughter I could eat any and everything. Once she was born I went back to being allergic. I am also allergic to some spices. I am not sure which ones and don't really want to know because I am a lover of food.

I have found that when I eat certain foods I tend to flare up more. Theses foods are caffeine, gluten and dairy. I replace my coffee with a peppermint ginger tea. I only use milk when I am cooking or baking. When I was younger I would drink milk all of the time. Morning and night. Now I can't even stomach a cup of milk. Gluten makes me feel sluggish and bloated.

There is no set diet plan to follow. I would recommend to eliminate one food at a time for 2 weeks and see how you feel. You can substitute it for a healthier choice or just eliminate it all together. For example instead having cake for a snack which contains gluten, dairy and sugar. You could have some grapes or a salad. Consult with your doctor or dietician.

I try my best to remain calm and peaceful. I think about what is going on to make me feel better altogether as one. Fibromyalgia is a systemic disease with multiple unknown causes. Treat it that way by treating your whole body.

Conclusion: Living With Fibromyalgia

Fibromyalgia is a beast. It is a chronic condition that I will have for the rest of my life. A disease that I have to deal with every single day. It doesn't matter where I am or what's going on, it can flare up at any given time. The trick is to not let it consume you and run your life.

I follow a daily routine that works for me. I was blessed to be able to have a job where I work remotely. For getting up at an early hour each morning results in me being tired leading to exhaustion. Then I have to fight with traffic to get to a job that is freezing cold in a building, where I can not control the temperature. While I sit upright or stand on my feet for hours. All while flaring up. How fair is that? Let's not forget that this is everyday. You would think that my body could only take so much.

However, I pull up my big girl panties and keep it moving. I don't have time to stop and let it all crash on me. The moment I give in, I may flare up for hours, days, weeks or months. Knock on wood I haven't had a flare up that lasts for months in a few years. They do last for days into weeks though. But, I believe I have a better hold onto this disease. It doesn't keep me down in the bed for to long. I am to cope with it. I am a functioning Fibromyalgia patient. It does not own me.

Fibromyalgia has taught me a lot. It has taught me patience. I cannot rush myself through a day nor life. I have to take it one step at a time. I know my body very well. I know how far I can push myself and my limits. I am not afraid to say no. Fibromyalgia has taught me to love myself for me. Flaws and all. I understand me. I know what hurts me and gives me peace. I am all about being painfree and peaceful. It is what I practice.

I appreciate each moment in life. Each experience and lesson. I try to capture my experiences and moments with loved ones. For as you know my memory, unfortunately is not the best. I love to remember the good times. Although the bad times have helped shaped me. Life's moments should not be taken in vain. It is precious and a gift.

I envy healthy people. They just don't know how good they have it. I wish I could just go off of four hours of sleep, junk food, physical contact, loud environment, over stimulating environments. And be just fine. So happy and full of energy. While I'm over here limited to one activity per week. So when I do get that burst of energy, I take full advantage of it. I try to do as much as I can do while pacing myself.

Sharing knowledge gained over the years has been my dream, and I have finally remembered to finish this book. It's ok, go ahead laugh. I did complete this project. For living with Fibromyalgia is doable.

Since my first encounter with fibromyalgia, the changes in treatments/products involved with this disease have been a slow process. There are tons of research and books on

Fibromyalgia. However, there are no real stories on how it actually feels. There is so much to tell. It feels like everything on your body hurts.

There are also no mention of what Fibromyalgia does to the relationship of the family and friends around you. You are in pain, but so are they. A strong support system goes a long way. But, you must keep in mind that this disease can also harm relationships. I have lost friends behind this disease. Some people just don't understand that each day you do not feel good. You just try to make the most out of it. Well at least I do. There will be people that get tired of hearing you complain. And then there will be people who don't believe that you are in the pain that you are in. Or will say oh I forgot that you hurting.

Sadly there are even doctors who won't believe you. I have had that before. A doctor told me that I wasn't feeling what I was feeling. Another physician perceived me as overexaggerating. Now if the doctors don't believe me. And the family thinks that I am seeking attention. Then what. Then I pray. God believes me and will provide me with relief as long as I keep on believing and fighting. Dealing with these issues is often too much for someone with severe fibromyalgia as they are too sick and cannot make proper decisions. I have my home setup that whether I am in my living room or bedroom. If need be I have medicine and a pillow available to provide comfort during the flare up. I also keep my heating pad near me. Along with keeping an icepack frozen at all times. I am always prepared for a flare up. I have things in place for any and all occasions and situations, where I will need relief. For Fibromyalgia does not run my life. I am always ready because this is real.

Research and networking with others who are living with fibromyalgia is a great way to find a support system. I find it soothing to talk to like minds. It let's me know that I am not alone. That there are others like me, that feels the same way that I feel. Fibromyalgia is not all up in my head. What I feel is real. What you are feeling is real. Do not let anyone tell you any different. Pain can not be measured.

Living with fibromyalgia is and will continue to be a challenge. Although today there are good options available for those who suffer from this disease. Sadly the many choices available that are prescribed has a lot of side effects. If we could get something that is friendly to the body and environment that would be ideal. For me the holistic approach has been safe.

Fibromyalgia is finally receiving needed attention from the public. As more research studies are being held. I hope that we get closer to a cure. It is not fair for anyone to have to suffer day in and out. I hope for relief for all chronic illnesses.